Sauna for Beginners

First Published in 2025
© Wolfbait Books
www.wolbait.co.uk

ISBN: 978-1-917298-10-0 (paperback)
ISBN: 978-1-917298-11-7 (ebook)

Illustrations by Colin Gordon
www.colingordon.net

All rights reserved. No part of this publication may be reproduced, stored in a retrieval system, or transmitted in any form or by any means — electronic, mechanical, photocopying, recording, or otherwise — without prior written permission from the copyright owners and publishers.

This book is intended as a general guide for personal use. The information provided is for reference only and should not be considered medical advice, diagnosis, or treatment. The author and publisher are not medical professionals or counsellors. Before beginning any health-related practice, consult a qualified professional.

A CIP catalogue record for this book is available from the British Library.

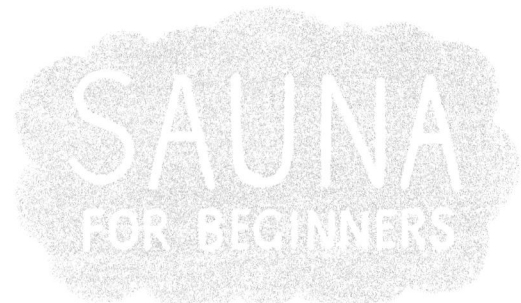

SAUNA FOR BEGINNERS

A Pocket Guide

By Yahya El-Droubie

Illustrations by Colin Gordon

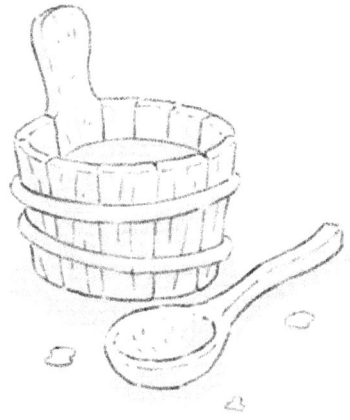

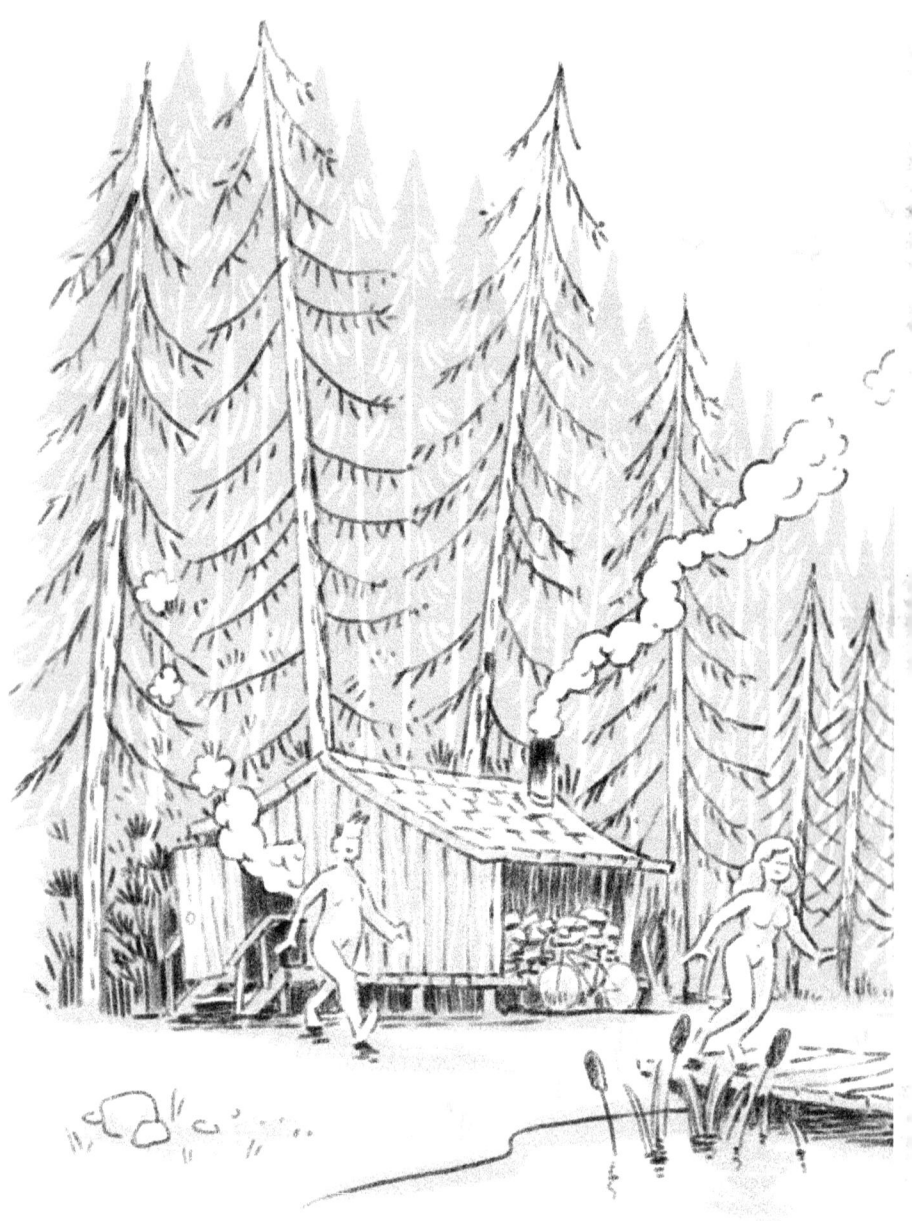

Contents

Introduction 7

Types of Heat Bathing 9

Health Benefits 11

Sauna Etiquette 14

Naked or Not? 19

Aufguss 22

Final Thoughts 22

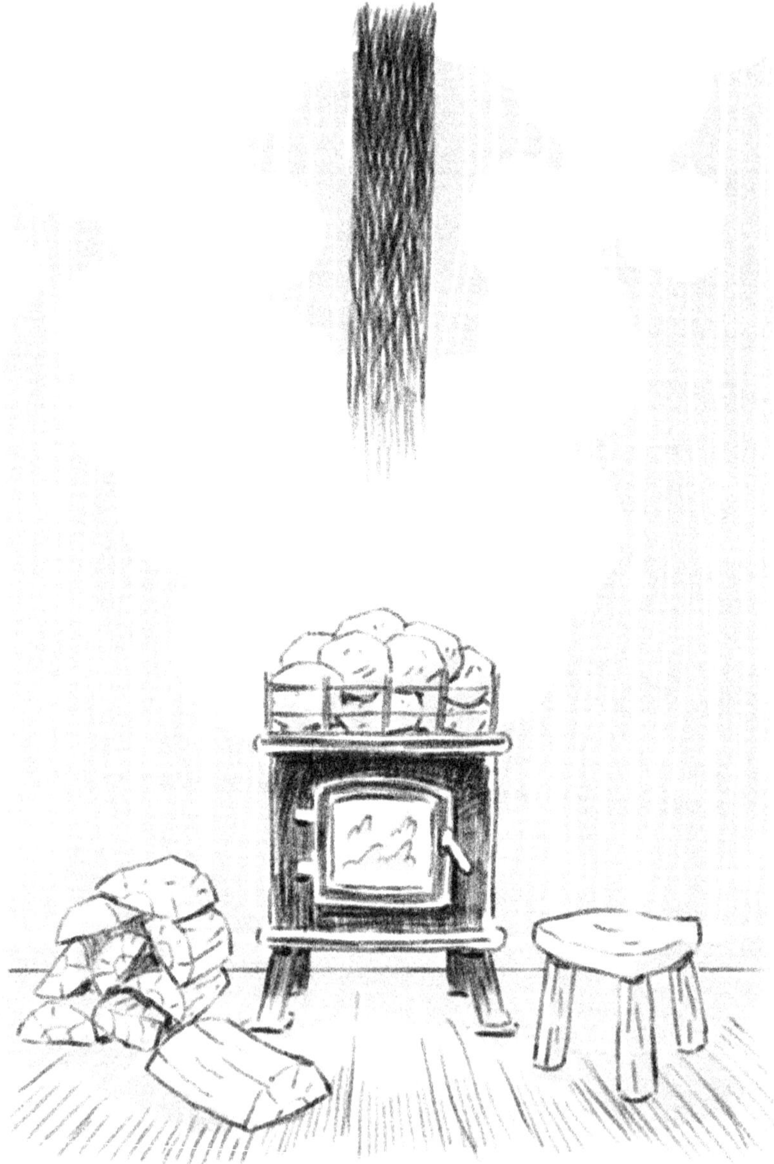

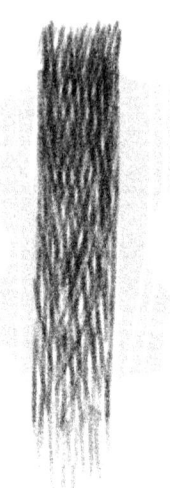

Introduction

SAUNAS ARE having a moment — they're officially on-trend. From converted horse boxes on beaches to chic rooftop spots in the city, people are finding new ways to sweat it out. And it's no longer just about the heat — the sauna has evolved into a space to unplug, connect with others, and recharge.

What's remarkable is the blending of traditional and modern practices. Sure, the Finns and Russians have been doing this forever, but now, countries without a long sauna tradition are adding their own unique spin. No fixed rules, just good vibes. Perhaps that's why saunas are becoming the new social hotspots — like pubs and bars, but without the hangover.

Many saunas, especially in Nordic countries, are tucked away in forests or perched beside lakes. It's about reconnecting with nature and the elements as well as your body. There's something magical about stepping out of a hot sauna and into the crisp air, surrounded by nothing but trees and sky. Sauna and wild swimming go hand in hand, whether it's plunging into a lake in the summer or diving into a hole carved out of ice in winter.

This guide explores sauna and other types of heat bathing, looking at their numerous benefits to physical and mental health, and revealing everything you need to know about sauna etiquette.

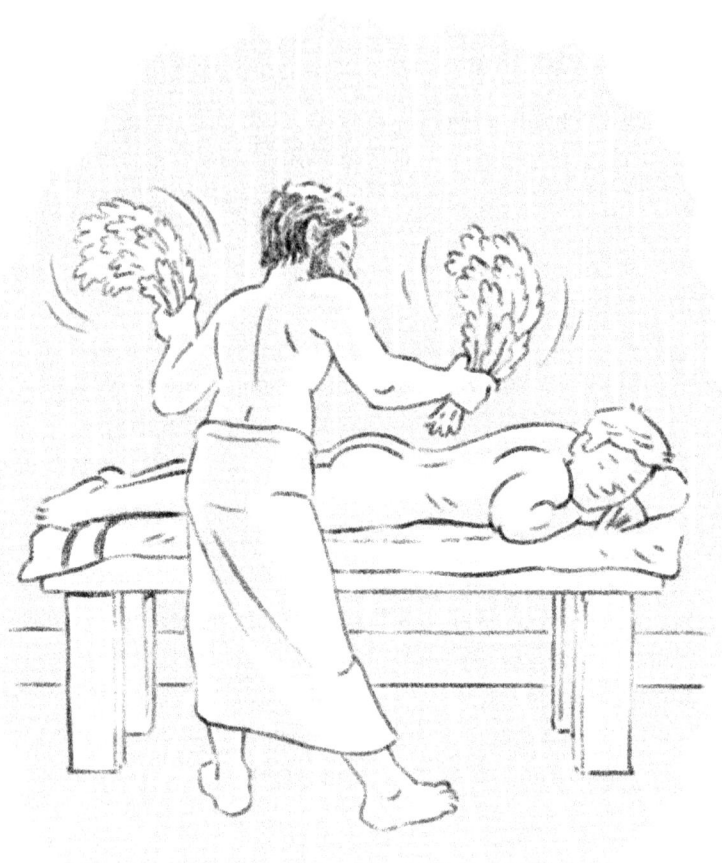

Types of Heat Bathing

MANY CULTURES around the world have heat bathing traditions. From steamy to super-hot, here's an overview of the best known types.

Traditional Finnish Sauna
The classic wood-lined room with a pile of hot stones. This is what most people think of when they hear the word "sauna". Heat comes from either an electric heater or a wood-burning stove, and the stones can be splashed with water to create steam. Temperatures usually hit 80–100°C (175–212°F).

Russian Banya
Think of this Slavic bathhouse as the Finnish sauna's more intense cousin. The banya gets seriously hot (up to 100°C/212°F) and steamy, and the signature experience is being whipped with a venik — a fragrant bundle of leafy branches, typically made from birch or oak, to boost circulation. Sounds weird, feels amazing! Between heat sessions, you'll often find people diving into ice-cold pools or rolling in the snow. It's a social thing, too — many see the banya as the perfect place to relax with friends and have a drink.

Infrared Sauna
The new kid on the block. Instead of heating the air, infrared lamps warm the body directly. The temperature runs cooler than a tradtional sauna (around 50–65°C/120–150°F), but you'll still break a good sweat. Great for people who find traditional saunas too intense.

Steam Room (Hammam)

The Turkish hammam is the classic steam bath — a tiled room filled with wet heat (100 per cent humidity) at lower temperatures (around 40°C/104°F). The hammam is far more humid than a traditional sauna. Often, the experience will include a massage or body scrub. You'll find similar steam rooms in many modern spas, though usually without the full traditional service.

Korean Jjimjilbang

These are full-service bathhouses with different specialised heated rooms. You might find rooms lined with jade, salt, clay, or minerals, each offering a different temperature and experience. Jjimjilbangs are much more than just a sauna: people spend hours here, moving between hot and cold rooms, getting scrubs, eating in the communal area, and even napping. They are a social hangout and wellness spot rolled into one. Some jjimjilbangs are open 24 hours, making them a great way to end a night out.

Japanese Onsen

While not technically a sauna, these natural hot spring baths are Japan's contribution to heat bathing culture. Usually very hot (around 40–44°C/104–111°F) and with mineral-rich water, they often have both indoor and outdoor pools with stunning views. Like the Finnish sauna, the onsen is traditionally enjoyed nude, with a focus on cleanliness and relaxation.

Modern Spa Mix

Many modern spas offer a variety of these heat bathing traditions. You might find a Finnish sauna next to a steam room, with a cold plunge and a relaxation area nearby. It's a great way to experience different heat bathing styles and discover what works best for you.

Health Benefits

Combining the heat of sauna with the shock of cold exposure provides a potent blend of health benefits that go beyond those offered by each practice individually, enhancing our well-being in several key ways.

Heart Health
The sauna gets the heart pumping, much like moderate exercise. Heat exposure increases the heart rate and opens up blood vessels, improving circulation. When you follow a sauna session with cold exposure, such as a cold plunge, those blood vessels quickly contract, creating a natural pumping effect that helps them become more flexible and responsive.

Recovery and Performance
The combination of heat and cold significantly aids recovery from exercise. The sauna's heat relaxes the muscles and increases blood flow, while cold exposure reduces inflammation and soreness. This makes it particularly effective after workouts, helping to reduce muscle strain.

Immune System
Alternating between heat and cold helps boost the immune system. The sauna's heat mimics a fever, stimulating immune function, while cold exposure increases white blood cells and reduces inflammation. This combination helps the body fight off illness more effectively.

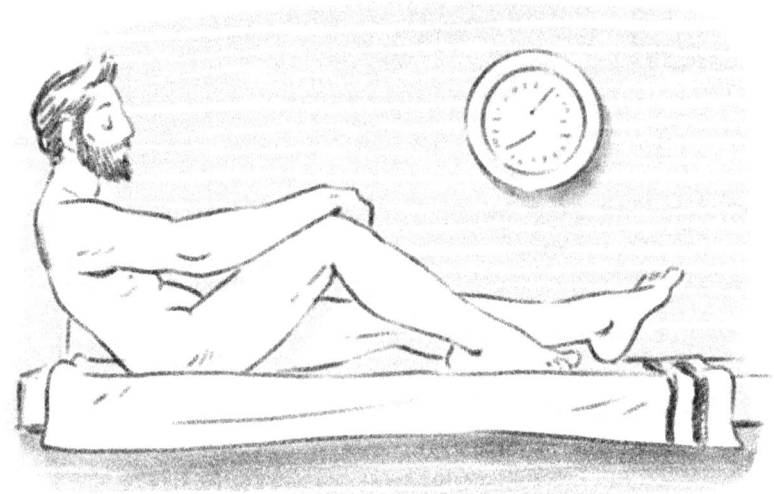

Mental Well-being

Moving between heat and cold has notable effects on our mental state. The hot sauna promotes relaxation and triggers the release of feelgood endorphins, while the cold plunge stimulates norepinephrine, which can improve focus and mood. Regular practice reduces stress and boosts mental clarity.

Metabolism

Heat exposure increases our metabolic rate through temperature stress, while cold activates calorie burning to generate warmth. This combination can support healthy weight management and metabolic function.

Sleep

Many find that regular sauna use improves their sleep. The temperature changes help regulate the body's core temperature and circadian rhythms. If you're looking for better sleep, try having a sauna 2–3 hours before bedtime.

Stress Reduction

Regular sauna sessions can help reduce levels of the stress hormone cortisol, allowing the body and mind to better adapt to various stressors. It's a simple but effective way to build our physical and mental resilience.

Safety

If you have heart problems or high blood pressure, check with your doctor beforehand. Don't use the sauna or cold plunge after drinking alcohol, and be sure to stay hydrated throughout a session.

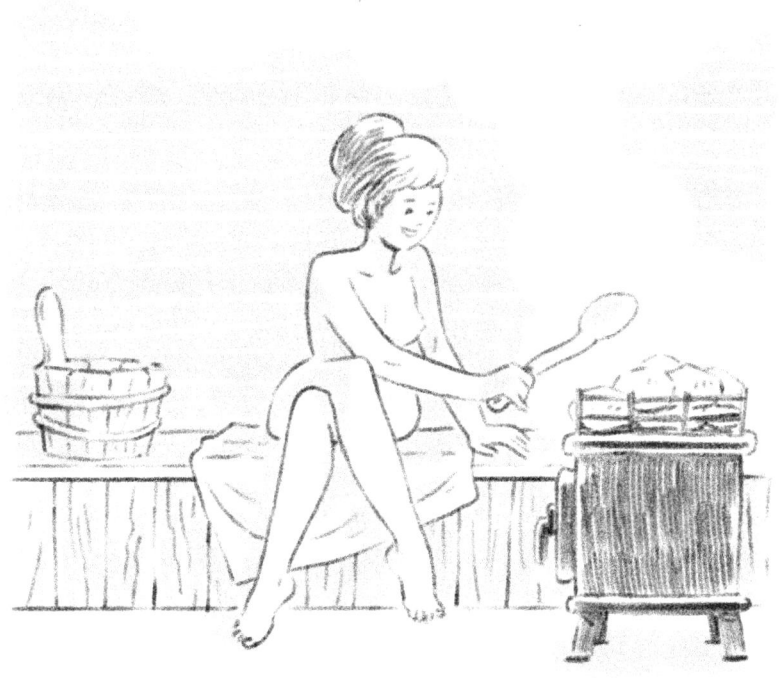

Sauna Etiquette

THE SAUNA should be your happy place — a retreat from the chaos of the world outside. Here are a few basic guidelines to help keep it that way.

What to Bring (And What to Leave Behind)

Before heading to the sauna, remove all jewellery and metal accessories — they can get uncomfortably hot and potentially burn your skin. And as heat will open your pores, it's best to remove makeup and skincare products too.

Pack at least two towels – one to sit on in the sauna and another for drying off afterwards. Some people swear by Turkish towels (peshtemals) — they're thin, absorbent, and dry super fast. Those thick, fluffy bathroom towels might feel luxurious, but they'll get heavy when wet and take forever to dry between rounds.

You might want to bring a water bottle, but don't take it into the sauna. Plastic and heat aren't a good mix, and metal and glass bottles can become dangerously hot. One last thing: don't forget your flip-flops.

Ditch the Phone

Let's be honest, your phone doesn't belong in the sauna. The heat and steam will probably kill it (and no, that waterproof rating won't protect it). Plus, nobody wants to see your glowing screen while they're trying to Zen out. Do yourself a favour — leave your phone in your locker and disconnect.

Choose the Right Outfit

To reap the full health benefits of your sauna experience, the best "outfit" to wear is your birthday suit (see pages 19–21). However, if the sauna you're visiting isn't textile free, try to avoid clothing that might trap sweat or chemicals against your skin. Linen shorts are a great substitute for trunks — linen is a natural fibre that allows the skin to breathe; it also absorbs moisture and will keep you comfortable while you're cooling off. Also consider wearing a sauna hat. This traditional accessory, typically made from felt, helps regulate temperature by protecting the head from excessive heat.

Shower First

Before you head into the sauna, take a quick shower. This rinses off sweat, dirt, and bacteria, and also helps keep the sauna clean for others. Leave the grime from the outside world outside! If you've been swimming in a pool, it's especially important to shower, because chlorine doesn't mix well with heat.

Enter/Exit the Sauna Quickly

Avoid leaving the door ajar for too long when entering or exiting, as it will lower the temperature and allow steam to escape. And nobody likes a draught. If you're stepping out to cool down and re-entering, that's totally fine — just be sure to close the door behind you to keep the heat in.

Go Barefoot

When you enter the sauna, it's best to leave your footwear outside. You don't want to bring in dirt on the soles of your flip-flops. And don't leave them cluttering up the doorway — saunas are often small, and nobody wants to trip over your footwear.

Sit on a Towel

Once inside the sauna, always sit on a towel — especially if you're not wearing a swimsuit. It's just good hygiene. Nobody wants to sit in a puddle of your sweat after you leave! Plus, it helps protect the wood. In countries like Germany, it's common practice to also have your feet on your towel.

Respect Personal Space

It's easy to get comfortable in a sauna, but be mindful of personal space when others are around. Spreading out too much can make people feel uncomfortable, especially if they're too polite or shy to ask you to move. If the sauna is busy, avoid lying down.

Don't Apply Water Without Asking

Always ask other sauna users before pouring water on the hot stones as the surge in humidity and temperature can be uncomfortable or even overwhelming for some. If they agree, use the ladle to pour small amounts of water at a time rather than dumping a large quantity at once.

Be Aware of Group Dynamics

Keep conversation quiet and relaxed — the sauna is for unwinding, not networking or heated debates. If others are keeping quiet, follow their lead. Be mindful of how much space you're taking up and how loud your voice is.

Time Your Sauna Session Right

A typical sauna round lasts 15–20 minutes, often followed by 1–2 minutes in the cold plunge. If you're a beginner, start with shorter times and gradually build up as your body adapts. You can repeat this process 2–3 times per session. Always listen to your body and avoid pushing it too hard. Remember, sauna time should be enjoyable, not an endurance test.

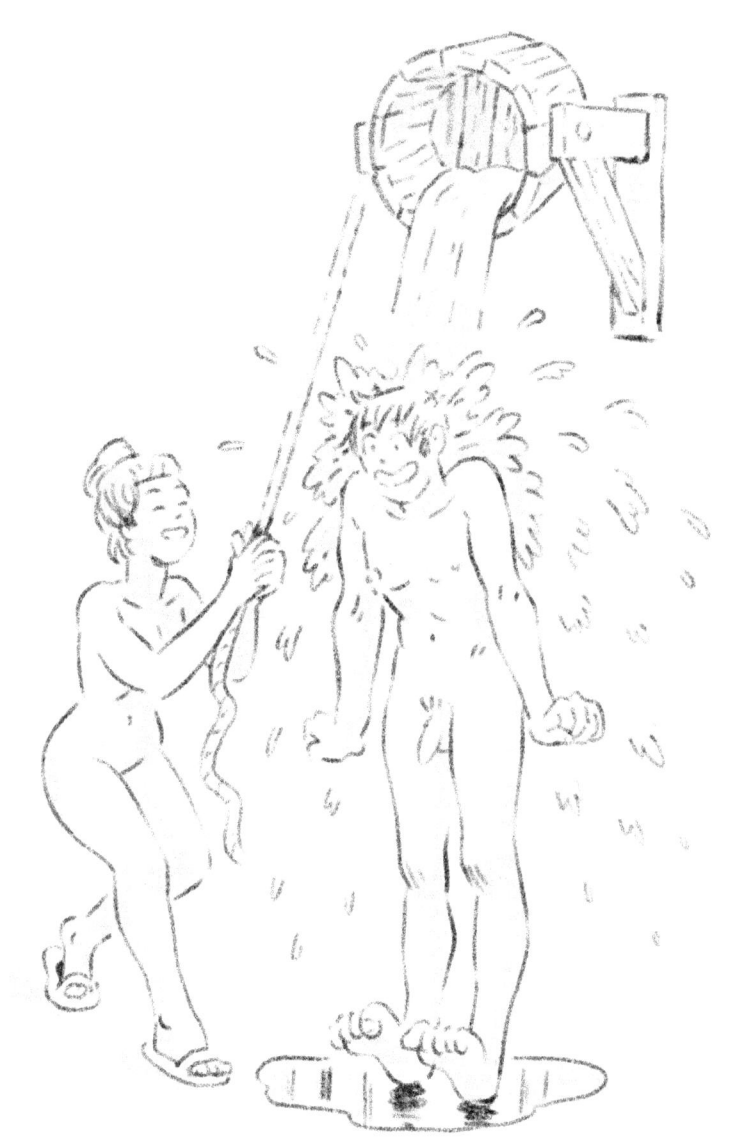

Cool Down Properly

Take your time to cool off. After each sauna round, allow 5–10 minutes for your body to return to normal temperature. Cooling down prevents overheating. Jump into the cold plunge or take a refreshing dip in the sea to boost circulation and help your body reset before heading back in!

At some saunas, you'll find a wooden bucket filled with cold water attached to the wall. The bucket usually has a chain or rope and can be toppled so the water is poured — or dumped — over you in one go. It's incredibly invigorating and will take your sauna experience to the next level.

Maximise Your Comfort

Following good sauna etiquette ensures a comfortable experience for everyone, but there's one question that often lingers: should you go nude? Sauna culture varies worldwide, and whether to strip down or cover up can depend on tradition, location, and personal comfort. Let's explore the ins and outs of going bare — and why it might not be as intimidating as you think.

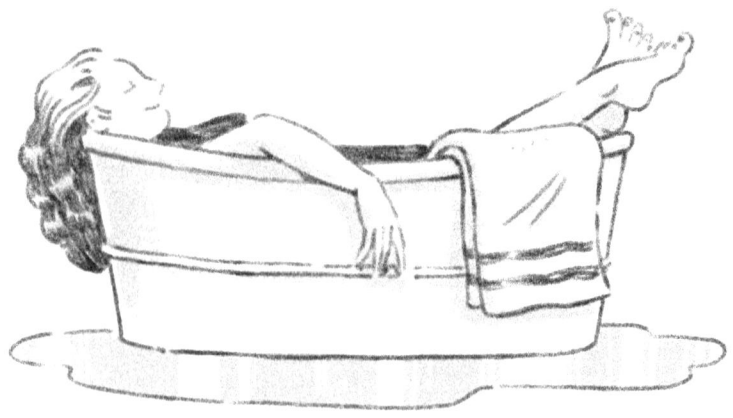

Naked or Not?

WHILE CULTURAL norms and personal preferences will often dictate what clothing to wear to get the most out of your sauna experience it's highly recommended that you strip off. There are numerous advantages to using a sauna in the nude, from the physiological to the psychological and even the social.

Physical Benefits of Going Nude

The most compelling reason to sauna nude is to maximise the health benefits. The primary purpose of a sauna is to induce sweating through heat exposure, and clothing creates an unwanted barrier to this process. When clothes trap sweat against your skin, they can restrict the natural evaporation process, potentially leading to irritation or rashes, particularly with synthetic materials. Being nude allows your skin — the body's largest organ — to breathe and sweat freely, promoting better temperature regulation and circulation.

The Hazards of Swimwear

Most swimwear is made from synthetic materials — essentially, plastics — that can degrade in the intense heat of a sauna, potentially releasing small amounts of chemicals. Additionally, swimwear often contains traces of washing detergent, and if it has been worn in a pool, chlorine and other chemicals will also linger in the fibres. In the heat of the sauna, these substances can evaporate into the air and onto your skin. With your pores open from the high temperature, your body may absorb this unwanted cocktail of chemicals — precisely when you're trying to detox.

Social Benefits

Some facilities offer women-only or men-only sessions, while others are mixed-gender (often called "co-ed"). While single-gender environments have their place, it's in co-ed settings that the sauna experience truly shines, offering unique social and psychological benefits. A respectful, non-sexualised environment, where all body types and ages are accepted as natural, can be transformative for our body image and social attitudes. It's one of the few spaces where social barriers fall away, allowing people to just be themselves, regardless of gender, sexual orientation, or age. Many find that this mixed environment helps challenge and heal unhealthy cultural attitudes.

Mixed sessions are also great if you want to enjoy the sauna with your partner, friends, or family, regardless of who they are. If you prefer single-gender sessions, check the facility's schedule — many places alternate between different options throughout the week.

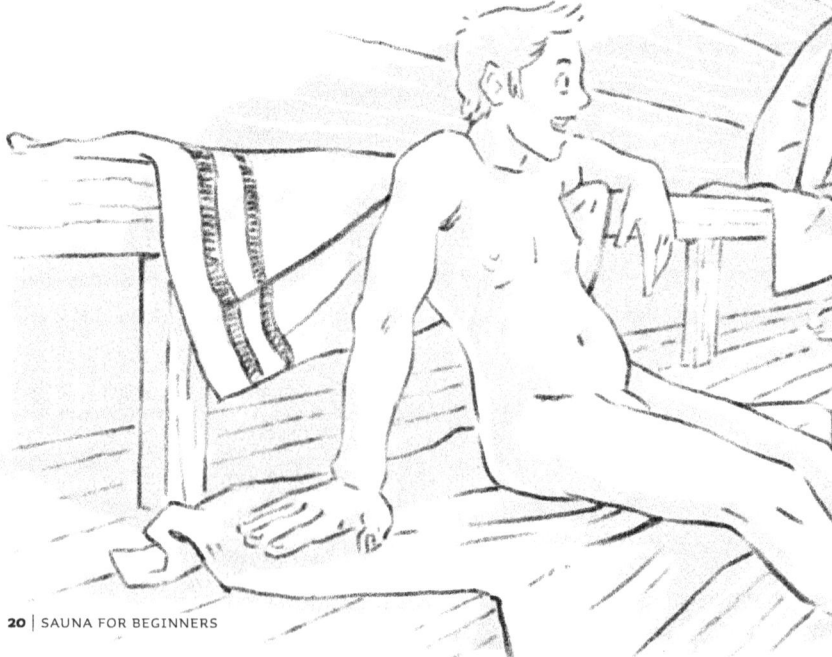

Making Your Choice

Nude sauna bathing isn't for everyone, and that's okay. Personal comfort and cultural background play a big part in the decision. However, if you're open to it, the benefits of going nude are hard to ignore. Don't worry if it feels odd at first — before long, you'll wonder what all the fuss was about. When we're in the sauna detoxing, there's something deeply satisfying about having shed our clothing — as if it's symbolic of the social masks we wear and the cultural baggage we carry.

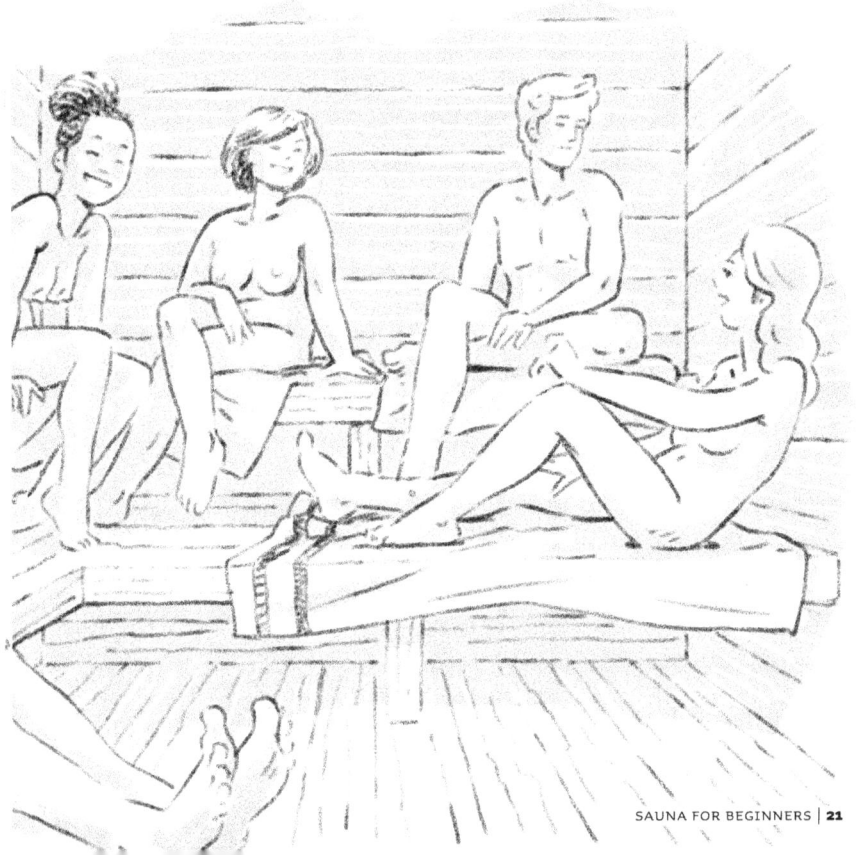

Aufguss

AUFGUSS IS a contemporary sauna ritual that transforms the simple act of adding water to hot stones into a multisensory theatrical experience. During the performance, specially prepared ice balls infused with essential oils are placed on the hot stones, releasing waves of fragrant steam as they melt. An Aufgussmeister will then use choreographed towel movements to circulate the steam and heat throughout the sauna. They'll often enhance the atmosphere with music and lighting effects. A typical session lasts 8–12 minutes and temperatures can reach 90°C/194°F. While intense, aufguss is one of the most entertaining ways to enliven your visit to the sauna.

Final Thoughts

WHETHER YOU'RE new to sauna or a seasoned enthusiast, the journey to relaxation, detoxification, and self-care can be incredibly rewarding. From the heat to the cold, the solitude to the social experience, saunas offer a space to reset, recharge, and reconnect with both your body and mind.

So, next time you step into a sauna, strip away your worries, embrace the heat, and allow yourself to fully experience the many benefits this tradition has to offer. You may just find that it's not only your body that feels rejuvenated, but your entire outlook on life.

Happy sweating!

www.ingramcontent.com/pod-product-compliance
Lightning Source LLC
Chambersburg PA
CBHW020029040426
42333CB00039B/865